The 3 Keys To Massive Weight Loss

(the right approach)

The Absolute Strategy To Eradicating Excess Fat

Godsend Morgan

All rights reserved. No part of this publication may be reproduced, distributed or transmitted in any form or by any means, including photocopying, recording, or other electronic or mechanical methods, without the prior written permission of the publisher, except in case of brief quotations embodied in critical reviews and certain other non-commercial uses permitted by Copyright law.

Copyright © by Godsend Morgan 2022

Contents

Introduction

Corpulence is pandemic in the US. The quantity of corpulent Americans has developed at an upsetting rate. Particularly throughout recent years, to the place where today a larger number of Americans are overweight than ordinary weight.

It currently viewed North by a little over half of Americans as overweight, with more than 30% of the populace viewed as corpulent (e.g., overweight by more than 20-30% of suggested weight).

These numbers portray a terrible general well-being circumstance. Being overweight builds an individual's gamble on a difficult disease.

An exceptionally enormous (and developing) level of residents are at expanded risk for creating serious ongoing infections, and face the possibility of early handicap or passing as the consequence of being overweight. In the discontinuity, the whole community strives. The weight of the subsequent expansion in medical care costs.

This book concerns weight reduction, an issue never internal to many individuals' psyches. Almost everybody needs to be thin and conditioned.

However, actually, it is far more straightforward to put on weight than to lose it. In the accompanying pages, the reasons for weight gain are surveyed, alongside various motivations behind why individuals ought to dedicate the work important to decrease their weight, to suggested levels. Having given inspiration to a health improvement plan, we close with a review of weight reduction techniques and ideas to accomplish long-lasting sound weight reduction.

Get everything rolling presently by turning the page.

Chapter 1

OBESITY AN EPIDERMIC

There are significant contrasts in wording that warrant note here. Medicalised accounts will generally utilize the terms stoutness. What's more overweight since these terms allude not exclusively to the size of a body, yet additionally that it is sick or at expanded risk of infection. Basic work, like that inside this unique version, problematizes the utilization of these terms, and where we use them here, we do as such with alert - utilizing them when we are alluding to scholastic or strategy work which marks bodies thusly, or on the other hand parts of sociology that challenge corpulence science in its specific manner. We are incredulous by these biomedical terms and the pathologization of bodies based on size. All the more frequently inside the sociologies the term 'fat' is utilized by journalists to limit any association with biomedical classes and for fat activists, it is utilized as a feature of a political system to recover the word, changing it into a marker of pride consequently countering its utilization to trash specific bodies.

The corpulence scourge in the US proceeds. Over the most recent couple of years, corpulence rates have not expanded fundamentally in a few US subpopulations, yet it is too early to let us whether know this implies that the scourge has arrived at the most extreme levels in these populaces 1, 2. There is obvious proof that weight rates are expanding in a significant part of the remainder of the world 3, 4. An enormous measure of examination is currently coordinated toward better comprehension and treatment of weight, and significant general well-being endeavors are coordinated toward decreasing stoutness rates. Until now, in any case, there is little proof of progress in switching the pestilence in the US.

Never to stress over the arrangement is here in this 3 strong key to tremendous poo in weight. The fact that obesity can be makes it very certain ninety percent switched, all that is needed is devotion and assurance.

Chapter 2

CAUSES OF OBESITY

Before looking into these 3 keys, is great you know and comprehend what the reason for weight is and how to defeat it for good.

Weight is by and large brought about by eating excessively and moving close to nothing. If you consume high measures of energy, especially fat and sugars, but don't consume practice and physical movement, a significant part of the excess energy will be put away by the body as fat.

Heftiness is for the most part brought about by eating excessively and moving pretty much nothing.

CALORIES

The energy worth of food is assessed in units called calories. The typical truly dynamic man needs around 2,500 calories per day to keep a sound weight, and the typical truly dynamic lady needs around 2,000 calories per day. This measure of calories may sound high, yet it very well may be not difficult to reach assuming you eat particular sorts of food. For instance, eating a huge focal point burger, fries, and a milkshake can add up to 1,500 calories and that is only 1 dinner.

Another issue is that many individuals are not genuinely dynamic, so loads of the calories they consume turn out to be put away in their bodies as fat.

POOR DIET

Stoutness doesn't work out pretty much by accident. It grows slowly over the long run, because of terrible eating routine and way of life decisions, for example:

1. Eating a lot of handled or cheap food - that is high in fat and sugar.
2. Drinking a lot of liquor - liquor contains a ton of calories, and individuals who drink intensely are much of the time overweight.
3. Eating out a ton - you might be enticed to likewise have a starter or pastry in a café, and the food can be higher in fat and sugar.
4. Eating bigger segments than you really want - you might be urged to eat excessively assuming your companions or family members are likewise eating huge parts.
5. Drinking such a large number of sweet beverages - including sodas and organic product juice.
6. Solace eating - assuming that you have low confidence or feel discouraged, you might eat to encourage yourself.

Undesirable dietary patterns will quite often run in families. You might advance terrible dietary patterns from your folks when you're youthful and proceed with them into adulthood.

Subsequently eating less immersed fat is exceptionally encouraged.

LACK OF PHYSICAL ACTIVITIES

The absence of active work is one more significant element connected with corpulence. Many individuals have occupations that include sitting in a work area for a large portion of the day. They likewise depend on their vehicles, instead of strolling or cycling. For unwinding, many individuals will quite often sit in front of the TV, peruse the web or play PC games, and seldom take customary activity.

On the off chance that you're not sufficiently dynamic, you don't utilize the energy given by the food you eat, and the additional energy you consume is put away by the body as fat.

The Department of Health and Social Care suggests that grown-ups do somewhere around 150 minutes of moderate-force vigorous movement, like cycling or quick strolling, consistently. This needn't bother with to be done all in a solitary meeting, yet can be separated into more modest periods. For instance, you could practice for 30 minutes per day for 5 days every week.

On the off chance that you're hefty and attempting to shed pounds, you might have to do more activity than this. It might assist with getting going gradually and steadily increment how much activity you do every week.

Subsequently, it is profoundly prompted that active work for grown-ups ought not to be ignored.

GENETICS

Certain individuals guarantee there's no good reason for attempting to get thinner since "it runs in my loved ones" or "it's in my qualities".

While there are a few uncommon hereditary circumstances that can cause corpulence, like Prader-Willi disorder, there's no great explanation why the vast majority can't get more fit?

The facts may demonstrate that specific hereditary qualities acquired from your folks, for example, having a huge hunger might make getting thinner is more troublesome, yet it positively doesn't make it unthinkable.

By and large, weight is more to do with ecological elements, for example, unfortunate dietary patterns got the hang of during adolescence.

Chapter 3

THE 3 KEYS TO MASSIVE WEIGHT LOSS

There are various ways of losing weight. With no further say or do we will be investigating these five discharges to gigantic weight reduction.

1. INTERMITTENT FASTING

One procedure that has become famous as of late is called irregular fasting. Discontinuous fasting is an eating design that includes standard, transient diets or times of negligible or no food utilization. The vast majority grasps discontinuous fasting as a weight reduction intercession. Fasting for brief timeframes assists individuals with eating fewer calories, which might bring about weight reduction over the long haul.

Be that as it may, irregular fasting may likewise assist with changing gamble factors for ailments like diabetes and cardiovascular illness, for example, bringing down cholesterol and glucose levels.

Choosing your intermittent fasting plan

There are a few different irregular fasting strategies. The most famous ones include:

    i. the 5:2 eating regimen

ii. the 16:8 technique

iii.   the Warrior diet

iv.   substitute day fasting (SDF)

v. Eat Stop Eat

All techniques can be successful. In any case, figuring out which one works best depends upon the individual.

To assist you with picking the strategy that accommodates your way of life, here's a breakdown of the upsides and downsides of each.

The 5:2 eating regimen

The 5:2 eating regimen is a clear discontinuous fasting plan.

Five days out of each week, you eat typically and don't confine calories. Then, at that point, on the other two days of the week, you decrease your calorie admission to one-fourth of your day-to-day needs. For somebody who routinely consumes 2,000 calories each day, this would mean diminishing their calorie consumption to only 500 calories each day, two days a week.

As indicated by a 2018 study trusted Source, the 5:2 eating routine is similarly basically as powerful as everyday calorie limitation for weight reduction and blood glucose control among those with type 2 diabetes.

Another investigation discovered that the 5:2 eating routine was similarly just about as powerful as constant calorie limitation for both weight reduction and the counteraction of metabolic illnesses like coronary illness and diabetes.

The 5:2 eating regimen gives adaptability, as you get to pick which days you quick, and there are no principles concerning what or when to eat on non-light days.

All things considered, worth focusing on eating "typically" on non-light days doesn't give you a free pass to eat anything you desire.

Limiting yourself to only 500 calories each day is difficult, regardless of whether it's just for two days out of every week.

Besides, consuming a couple of calories might cause you to feel sick or weak.

The 5:2 eating routine can be successful, yet it's not a great fit for everybody. Converse with your primary care physician to check whether the 5:2 eating regimen might be right for you.

The 16/8 method

The 16/8 discontinuous fasting plan is one of the most famous styles of fasting for weight reduction.

The arrangement confines food utilization and calorie-containing refreshments to a set window of 8 hours out of every day. It requires avoiding sustenance for the overabundance 16 hours of the day. While different eating regimens can set severe standards and guidelines, the 16/8 technique depends on a period-limited taking care of (PLTCO) model and is more adaptable.

You can pick any 8-hour window to consume calories.

Certain individuals pick to skip breakfast and eat from early afternoon to 8 pm, while others try not to eat late and adhere to a 9 am to 5 pm timetable. Restricting the number of hours that you can eat during the day might assist you with shedding pounds and lower your pulse.

Research shows that time-limited taking care of examples like the 16/8 strategy might forestall hypertension and lessen the measure of food eaten, prompting weight reduction.

A recent report tracked down that when joined with opposition preparing, the 16/8 technique helped diminish fat mass and keep up with bulk in male members. A later report viewed that the 16/8 technique didn't disable additions in muscle or strength in ladies performing opposition preparing.

While the 16/8 technique can without much of a stretch fit into any way of life, certain individuals might find it trying to try not to eat for 16 hours in a row.

Moreover, eating an excessive number of bites or low-quality food during your 8-hour window can invalidate the constructive outcomes related to 16/8 irregular fasting.

Make certain to eat a reasonable eating routine including organic products, vegetables, entire grains, solid fats, and protein to expand the potential medical advantages of this eating regimen.

The Warrior diet
The Warrior Diet is an irregular fasting plan in light of the eating examples of old heroes.
Made in 2001 by Ori Hofmekler, the Warrior Diet is somewhat more limited than the 16:8 technique but less prohibitive than the Eat Fast Eat strategy.
It comprises eating very little for 20 hours during the day and afterward eating as much food as wanted all through a 4-hour window around evening time.
The Warrior Diet urges well-being food nuts to eat up unobtrusive amounts of dairy things, hard-gurgled eggs, and crude products of the soil, as well as non-calorie liquids during the 20-hour quick period.
After this 20-hour quick, individuals can eat anything they need for a 4-hour window, however, natural, solid, and natural food sources are suggested.
While there's no exploration of the Warrior Diet explicitly, human examinations demonstrate that time-limited dealing with cycles can provoke weight decrease.

Time-bound dealing with cycles could have a collection of other clinical benefits. Concentrates on a show that time-limited dealing with cycles can hinder diabetes, slow development, delay development, and augmentation of the future in rodents.

More examination is required on the Warrior Diet to comprehend its advantages for weight loss. The Warrior Complete diet might be challenging to follow, as it limits significant calorie utilization to only 4 hours out of each day. Overconsumption in the evening time is a typical test.

The Warrior Diet may likewise prompt scattered eating designs.

Substitute day fasting (SDF)

Substitute day fasting is a discontinuous fasting plan with a memorable simple design. On this eating routine, you are quick every other day yet can eat anything you desire on the non-fasting days.

A few variants of this diet embrace a "changed" fasting methodology that includes eating around 500 calories on fasting days. Notwithstanding, different adaptations dispense with calories out and out on fasting days.

Substitute day fasting has demonstrated weight reduction benefits. A randomized pilot concentrating on contrasting substitute day fasting with a day-to-day caloric limitation in grown-ups with weight found the two techniques to be similarly powerful for weight reduction.

Another investigation discovered that members consumed 35% fewer calories and lost a normal of 7.7 pounds

(3.5 kg) later switching back and forth between a day and a half of fasting and 12 hours of limitless eating north of about a month.

If you truly have any desire to augment weight reduction, adding an activity system to your life can help.

Research shows that consolidating substitute day fasting with perseverance exercise might cause two times as much weight reduction than just fasting. A full speedy every other day can be incredible, especially if you're new to fasting. Gorging on non-fasting days can likewise be enticing.

If you're new to irregular fasting, slide into substitute day fasting with a changed fasting plan.

Whether you start with a changed fasting plan or full quick, it's ideal to keep a nutritious eating regimen, consolidating high protein food varieties and low-calorie vegetables to assist you with feeling full.

Eat Stop Eat

Eat Stop Eat is a whimsical way to deal with discontinuous fasting promoted by Brad Pilon, writer of the book "Eat Stop Eat."

This irregular fasting plan includes recognizing a couple of non-continuous days out of every week during which you swear off eating, or quick, for a 24-hour time frame. During the excess days of the week, you can eat openly, yet it's prescribed to eat a balanced eating regimen and keep away from overconsumption. The reasoning behind a week after week 24-hour quick is that consuming fewer calories will prompt weight reduction.

Fasting for as long as 24 hours can prompt a metabolic shift that makes your body utilize fat as an energy source rather than glucose. Yet, keeping away from nourishment for 24 hours all at once requires a great deal of resolution and may prompt gorging and overconsumption later on.

It might likewise prompt confused eating designs.

More examination is required concerning the Eat Stop Eat diet to decide its potential medical advantages and weight reduction properties.

Converse with your Doctor before attempting Eat Stop Eat to check whether it could be a viable weight reduction answer for you.

How intermittent fasting affects your synthetic substances

Irregular fasting might assist you with shedding pounds, yet it can likewise influence your chemicals. That is because muscle-to-fat proportion is the body's way to deal with taking care of energy (calories).

At the point when you eat nothing, your body rolls out a few improvements to make it put away energy more open. Models remember changes in sensory system action, as well as significant changes in the levels of a few essential chemicals.

The following are two metabolic changes that happen when you quick:

i. Insulin

Insulin levels increment when you eat, and when you are quick, they decline decisively. Lower levels of insulin work with fat consumption.

ii. Norepinephrine (noradrenaline).

Your sensory system sends norepinephrine to your fat cells, making them separate muscle-to-fat ratio into free unsaturated fats that can be signed for energy.

Curiously, regardless of what a few defenders of consuming 5-6 dinners each day guarantee, momentary fasting might increment fat consumption.

Research shows that other day fasting preliminaries enduring 3-12 weeks, as well as entire day fasting preliminaries enduring 12-24 weeks, diminish body weight and muscle versus fat

Intermittent fasting assists you with diminishing calories and shed pounds

The primary explanation that discontinuous fasting works for weight reduction is that it assists you with eating fewer calories.

Every one of the various conventions includes skipping dinners during the fasting time frames

Except if you repay by eating substantially more during the eating time frame, you'll be consuming fewer calories. As indicated by a 2014 survey, irregular fasting decreased body weight by 3-8% over a time of 3-24 weeks.

While inspecting the pace of weight reduction, discontinuous fasting might deliver weight reduction at a pace of roughly 0.55 to 1.65 pounds (0.25-0.75 kg) each week.

Individuals likewise encountered a 4-7% decrease in midsection perimeter, showing that they lost tummy fat.

These outcomes show that discontinuous fasting can be a valuable weight reduction device.

2. DIET

Another strategy is dieting, the choice of food we eat has a very great impact on our health and most importantly on our weight.

This system help to regularize what we eat to support a beneficial outcome in achieving weight reduction.

Cut back on refined carbohydrates

One method for getting in shape rapidly is to scale back sugars and starches, or carbohydrates. This could be with a low-carbohydrate eating plan or by reducing refined carbohydrates and replacing them with whole grains

At the point when that's what you do, your craving levels go down, and you by and large wind up eating fewer calories. With a low-carbohydrate eating plan, you'll use consuming put away fat for energy rather than carbohydrates.

If you decide to eat more complicated carbohydrates like entire grains alongside a calorie deficiency, you'll profit from higher fiber and review them all the more leisurely. This makes them more filling to keep you content.

A recent report affirmed that an exceptionally low starch diet helped shed pounds in more established populations.

Research likewise proposes that a low-carbohydrate diet might decrease hunger, which can prompt normally eating fewer calories without even batting an eye or feeling hungry.

Note that the drawn-out impacts of a low-carbohydrate diet are as yet being explored. It can likewise be challenging to stick to a low-carbohydrate diet, which might prompt you to eat less junk food and have fewer outcomes in keeping a solid weight.

There are possible drawbacks to a low-carbohydrate diet that might lead you to an alternate technique. Decreased

calorie diets can likewise prompt weight reduction and are more straightforward to keep up with for longer periods.

If you decide on an eating routine zeroing in rather on entire grains over refined carbohydrates, a recent report related high entire grain consumption with lower weight index (LWI).

Eat protein, fat, and vegetables
Expect to incorporate various food sources at every dinner. To change your plate and help you with getting more accommodated your meals should include:
i. a protein source.
ii. Vegetables.
iii. Fat source.
Iv. a little piece of mind-boggling carbs, like entire grains.

Protein
Eating a prescribed measure of protein is vital to assist with saving your well-being and bulk while shedding pounds.
Confirmation suggests that eating adequate protein could improve cardio metabolic risk factors, cravings, and body weight.
By and large, a normal male necessity is around 56-91 grams each day, and the typical female requirement is 46-75 grams each day, however many variables impact protein needs.

Here are rules to unnecessarily help you with figuring out how much protein to eat without eating:

i. 1-1.2g/kg of body weight for people 65 and more prepared

ii. 0.8g/kg of body weigh
iii. 1.4-2g/kg of body weight for competitors.

Counting calories with sufficient protein may likewise assist you with decreasing desires and nibbling by aiding you to feel full and fulfilled.
Solid protein sources include:
i. **Meat**: hamburger, chicken, pork, and sheep
ii. **Endlessly fish**: shrimp, salmon, sardines, and trout
iii. **Eggs**
iv. **Plant**-based proteins: beans, vegetables, quinoa, tempeh.

Vegetables

Feel free to stack your plate with rich green vegetables. They're stacked with enhancements, and you can eat very gigantic totals without essentially extending calories and carbohydrates.
All vegetables are supplement-rich and good food sources to add to your eating regimen, however, a few vegetables, similar to potatoes, yams, winter squash, and corn, are higher in carbohydrates.
These vegetables are viewed as complicated carbs because they contain fiber, yet you might need to be

aware of serving size while adding these vegetables to your plate.

Vegetables to incorporate a greater amount of:

i. tomatoes
ii. Spinach
iii. Kale
iv. Brussels sprouts
v. cabbage
vi. Broccoli
vii. Swiss chard
viii. Lettuce
ix. Cucumber
x. cauliflower
xi. Peppers

Solid fats

Try not to fear eating fats.

Your body requires strong fats paying little heed to what eating plan you pick. Olive oil and avocado oil are uncommon choices for recalling your eating plan. Nuts, seeds, olives, and avocados are delectable and solid increments, too.

Various fats, for instance, spread and coconut oil should be used solely with some limitation due to their higher drenched fat substance.

3. MOVE YOUR BODY

Exercise can assist you with getting thinner all the more rapidly. Lifting loads has especially great advantages.

While you're striving to get fit and get in shape, you need a customary schedule that gives solid outcomes. Uplifting news: You don't have to turn into a jock;

Concentrates on the show that more limited times of activity are more successful for fat misfortune. Nevertheless, what kind of action consumes the most calories?

These activities for weight reduction will direct you to the correct course:

Cardio works out and will smash calories. Running on a treadmill will consume 25-39% greater calories than doing portable weight practices at a similar degree of effort, according to a new report in the Journal of Strength and Conditioning Research. The fact that combining cardio and strength presents in any defense, your smartest option for weight reduction a normal.

Assuming you're strolling or running frantically without the outcomes you're searching for, building muscle might be vital to moving the scale.

Why? Since muscles are metabolically dynamic, so they consume calories in any event, when you're not working out. To fit cardio exercises and strength preparation into your exercise, consider stretch preparation, which specialists say is one of the most amazing ways of consuming fat.

By lifting loads, you'll consume calories and help with holding your processing back from toning down, which is a normal consequence of getting more slender.

Attempt strength preparation three to four times each week. If you're new to lifting loads, a coach might have the option to assist you with a beginning. Guarantee your essential consideration doctor is furthermore aware of any new action plans

If lifting loads isn't a possibility for you, doing some cardio exercises like strolling, running, running, cycling, or swimming is exceptionally helpful for weight reduction and general well-being.

Both cardio and weightlifting might assist with weight reduction and deal with bunches of other medical advantages.

The advantages of span preparing

Sorting out in spans is one method for receiving the rewards of cardio and strength while boosting your calorie consumption in a short measure of time.

Stretch exercises include shifting back and forth between short explosions of extraordinary exertion and times of lower force or rest. The power resets your

Yet again processing to a higher rate during your activity, so it requires hours for your body to chill off. This's known as APOU (abundance post-practice oxygen utilization). That implies you consume calories long after you've

completed your exercise and thought about doing an exercise at a ceaseless moderate speed, as indicated by a recent report from the European Journal of Applied Physiology.

"Ranges are an extraordinary procedure for driving weight decline past the APOU impact. A great deal of weight reduction comes from the psychological side of the range additionally," says Chris Ryan, one of MIRROR's spreading out guides. "Ranges offer a stunning technique for harnessing individual success after every rep or round of activity, and not just viewing at the exercise in general."

To assist you with finding a calorie-consuming exercise that accommodates your way of life and objectives, we gathered together the best activities for weight reduction here.

Assuming that you're figuring out in spans, do the activity for 30 seconds consistently and rest for the excess 30 seconds. As you progress, you can expand your opportunity to 45 seconds of movement and 15 seconds of

rest. Keep in mind that you need to be working at your greatest, forgetting about your breath toward that span's end.

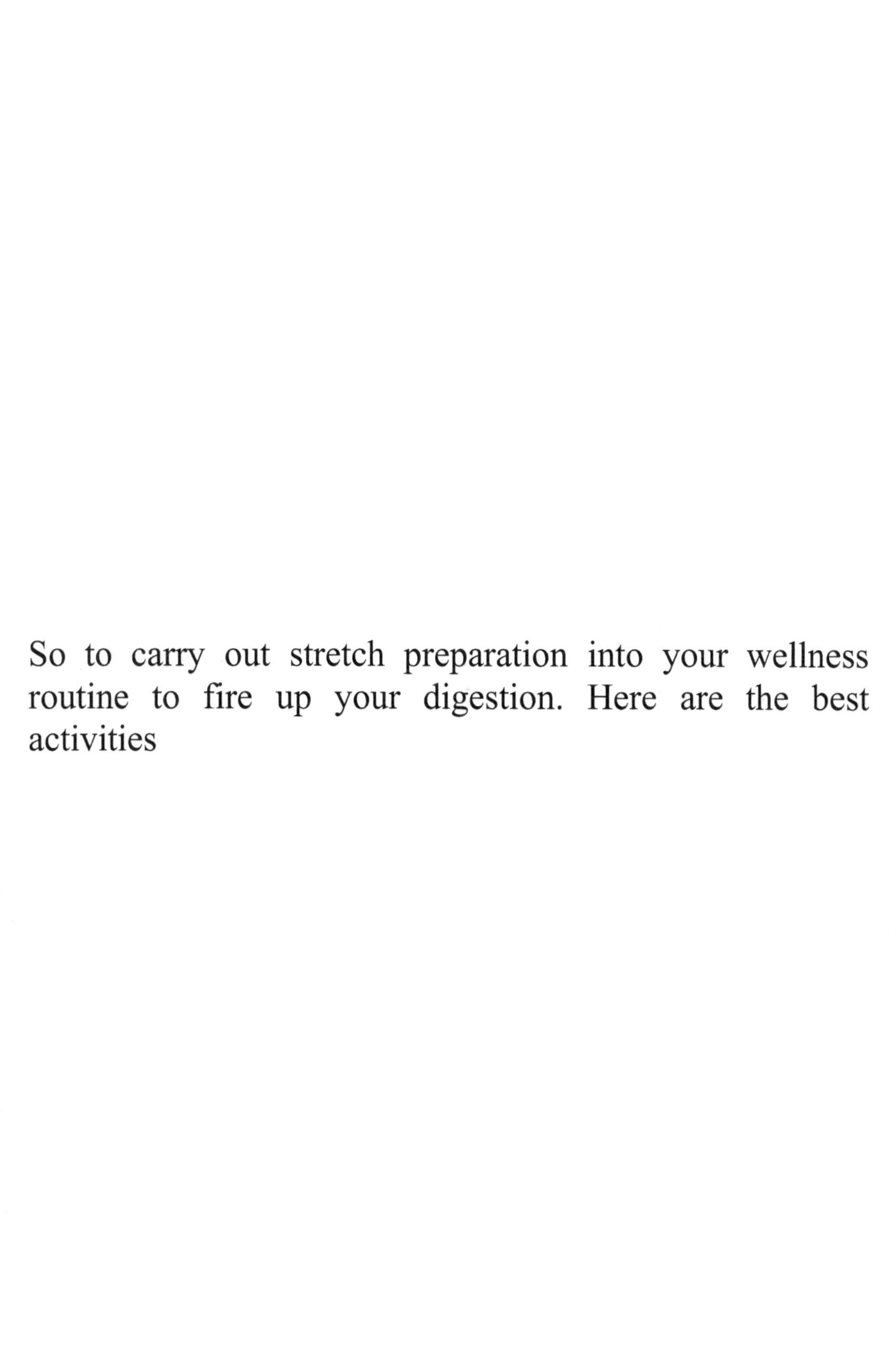

So to carry out stretch preparation into your wellness routine to fire up your digestion. Here are the best activities for weight reduction: Yoga, Swimming, Battle Ropes, Stairmaster, Rowing, Spinning, Kickboxing, Running, Jump, and so forth.

Chapter 4

CONCLUSION

It is vital to know which of these keys will be fitting for your timetable. Recollect not to surrender consistency is likewise an extremely fundamental device for accomplishing weight reduction. For fast impact, you can blend a movement from every one of the 3 keys referenced before. How about you start your process today stop the reasons, it's simply an issue of making a stride and you will see a monstrous change.

www.ingramcontent.com/pod-product-compliance
Lightning Source LLC
Chambersburg PA
CBHW070105260726
48658CB00002B/995